Karma Yoga and Mind

SANDEEP KHURANA

SANDEEP KHURANA

KARMA YOGA & MIND

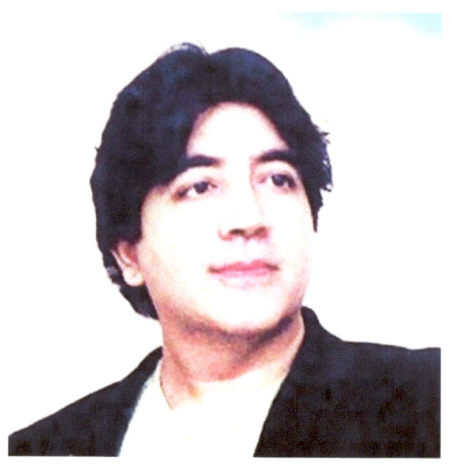

Sandeep Khurana is a spiritualist, writer, new age music composer and TV producer. He has written articles and produced films on Yoga, & Healing.

He has produced videos that have been aired on various TV channels in California, and his new age music in the categories of Yoga music, Relaxing music, sacred chants, healing music and fitness music, is in iTunes Top 100 New Age music charts. He has more than a million people in over 50 countries subscribing to his music. He has spent several years in studying various spiritual and healing methods, like Yoga, Reiki, Osho mysticism, Pranayama, Chakra healing and others. More information about his work in music and alternative healing is available on his websites

http://sandeepkhurana.com
http://skivamusic.com

Preface

Life with its infinite dimensions has always been a mystery to mankind in terms of what really determines its course of events, what exactly is the origin of thoughts, and what and why there is something that always goes on beyond the ordinary five senses. Interestingly, as linear time progresses, from generation to generation, century to century, from one age to another, the mystery deepens even more, leaving the entire humanity wondering and marveling at this intricate and supreme artwork from God called Life Experience. The limitations of human mind are unlimited, and life presents its complexities in infinite ways, whether it is to do with karmic associations, intricacies of events that happen, people playing numerous roles, and countless relationships one experiences on this planet. Yoga is about unification of mind with the higher mind, and hence the need to surrender to, 'Grace and Godliness' becomes unquestionably important. Trust on the instincts has to be complete in order to allow the healing to happen and allow the life to take its natural course.

Contents

Chapter 1: Thoughts & Healing

Thoughts engender healing, and the mind is always manufacturing thoughts constantly. However, the mystery behind thought creation and generation has been beyond our reach to completely comprehend. Thoughts owe their existence to opportunities, which are endless in time and space. Thoughts can be formed from telepathic interactions and soul communication between beings and entities. Karma, as an infinite process is continuously happening in the background, beyond human senses, and contributes to thought generation in many ways. Thoughts, as multidimensional energy beings have a life of their own. Their lifespan is determined by the truthfulness associated with those thoughts, the purity of intent and associated feelings that travels with them. Thoughts automatically become effective means of communication more than talking, writing, or using gestures. Those who attain spiritual awareness, after having worked for several years meditating, and following their soul path, begin to observe and manage their thoughts very well since they are aware of the potential the thought can have, and the manifestation, the thoughts are capable of bringing about.

SANDEEP KHURANA

Thoughts can relate to our past, originate or derive from our actions left incomplete, past hurts or joys, or can reveal themselves as messages and signals from the higher planes of existence. These planes are accessible to people who are clairvoyant, spiritually awakened and intuitive. The thoughts shimmering in various corners of the mind, if examined carefully, can help us point to the voids in the past, incomplete tasks we must complete, and the existing physical and mental pain situations that need to be healed. The energy body also contains such imprints, and energy healing and other alternative healing methods work on the subtle energy body to help get rid of past problematic situations. The voids also determine what path the person is likely to take in the future, and the actions, needed to balance those energy-voids. Tuning one's mind to the mind of another person for thought transmission and exchange opens new doors for healing and awakening. The subjects have to be willing to participate in the process to make it work. Techniques like meditation and yoga help one center one's mind and bring it to a state of 'thought stillness' to be able to communicate effectively over time and distance. The thought stillness places one in a state of surrender and prevents any ego to interfere with the process.

Awakened spiritual masters sitting miles away from one another can successfully exchange thoughts and use them for healing, communication and for the highest good of the universe.

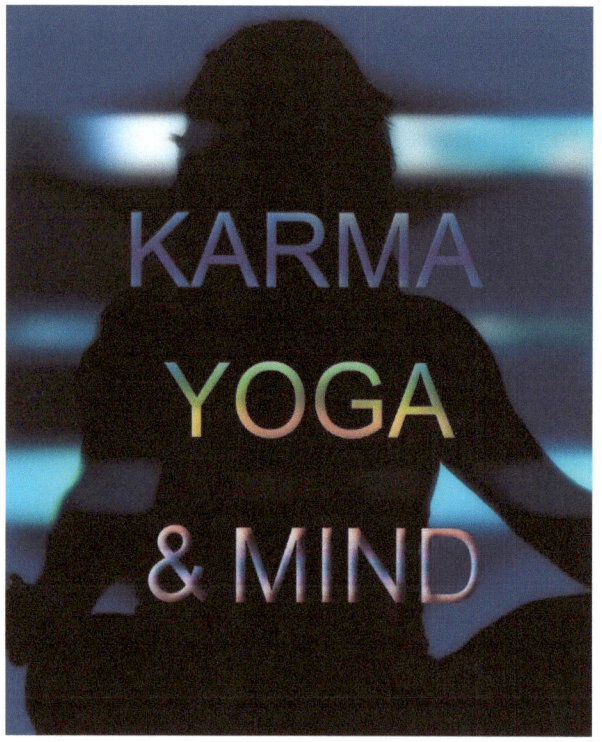

A big step towards enlightenment is following Yoga practices, using the power of mind, and dealing with Karma.

A major challenge in healing practice is dealing with our pre-existing beliefs and pre-conditioned mind. The mind tends to construct models of people and situations and we are persuaded to work with those models all our lives. Model is in this context is like a chain of thoughts integrated together as a belief or an interpretation or understanding of a life experience. We have our tendency to model things, event, people, and experiences, past, present and future. And then we have no other option but to operate on the basis of these models since they are deeply embedded in our thinking systems. These models blur our vision, sometimes significantly, and bring down our ability to see things clearly and distinctly. It is like looking at the world through a pair of self-prescribed glasses. As we continue to pile up and integrate these models all our lives, sometimes adding a predictive corrective approach, and sometimes even recreating the models after demolishing them partially or completely, our thought process and hence our life experience gets limited by the paradigms and beliefs that form the foundation of these models.

Change being a constant factor in life, this foundation is never steady, and changes with time and experience. Mind looks for constant stability in life which does not exist beyond theory. Every moment, millions of parameters are changing; new bonds form, older ones transform, and new beliefs manifest themselves. Yet the mind continues to interfere till it becomes powerless and surrenders to the soul or the inner self. The connection with inner self helps one to think beyond such models and static beliefs and be able to make life's decision better. This inner connection brings a healing power which begins to transform the life of the individual, directly working on root causes of physical and mental conditions. Over time the individual and the people around the individual begin to notice a significant positive change in the individual's behavior and way of life.

Chapter 2: Actions

Actions operate at a level that is beyond the level of thoughts. They are more tangible, more concrete, stronger as entities, and hence more irreversible so to say. Actions include speech. Actions have to be managed and monitored more carefully than thoughts, since they are likely to have higher impact in generating karmic influence and manifestation. There is an element of 'irreversible-ness' in thoughts, but less in actions, since actions are kind of thoughts implemented, or thoughts 'acted upon'. So a lot more care is needed in dealing with one's and other people's actions. It is interesting to have discovered how health situations can relate to our thoughts and actions. According to the studies in the spiritual sciences, we are much beyond and much more than a mere physical body.

The physical body is found to vibrate at the lower frequency in the energy world, and the next higher frequency than that of the physical body, is that of the etheric body which is like the life energy to the physical body. Beyond this, we have an astral body, mind body and then the causal body.

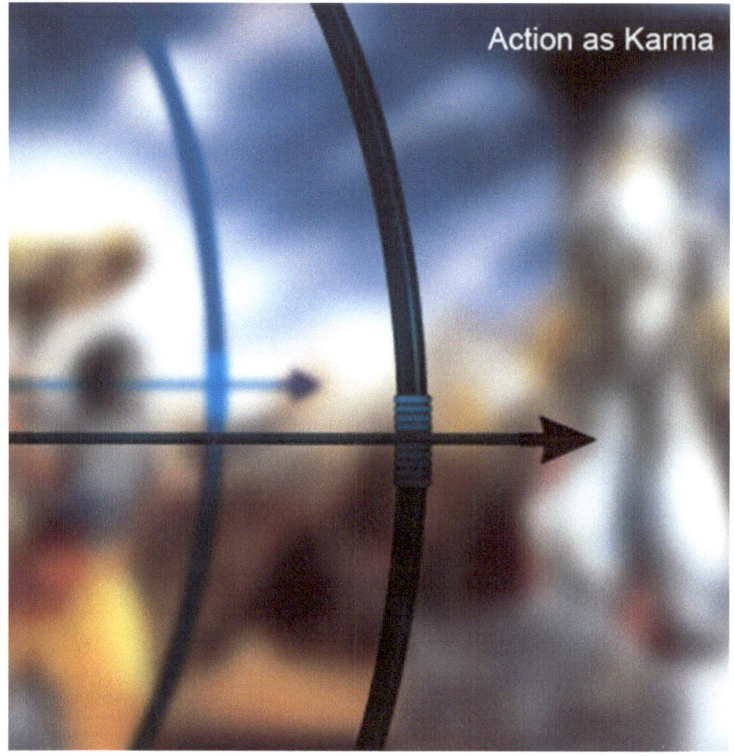

Karma or Action is based on Cause – Effect experience

Astral body is the energy body, the level at which we experience energy healing. Mind body transcends time and space, and engenders telepathic communication. Causal body helps us deal with past karmas, memories, and soul level vibrations.

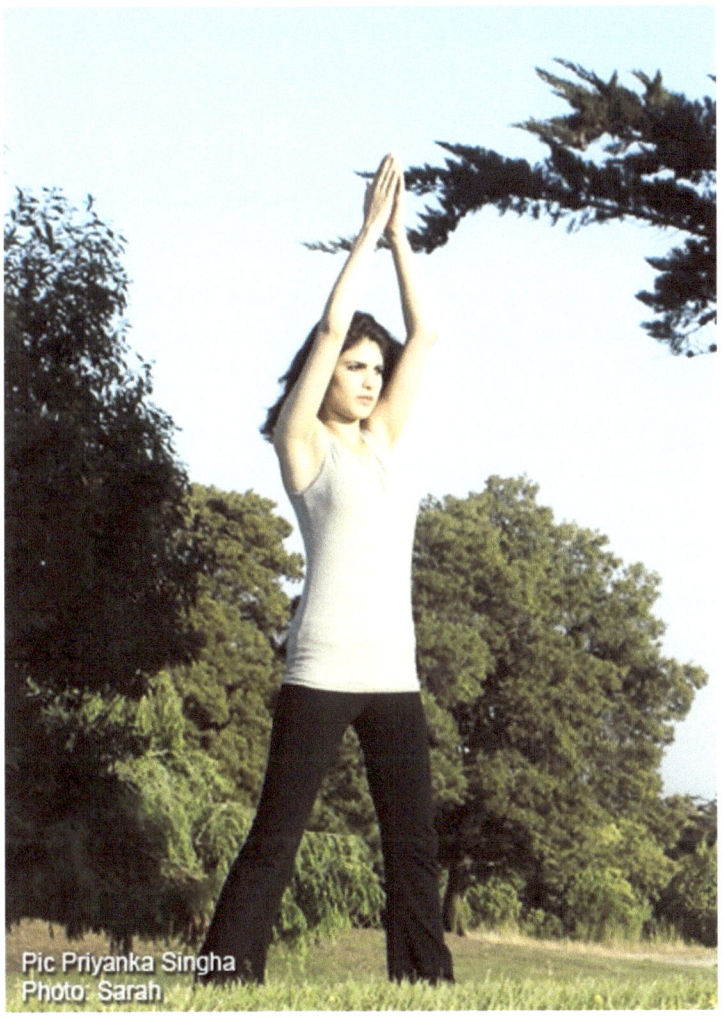

Pic Priyanka Singha
Photo: Sarah

As we become aware of the planes of existence that are beyond
the physical realm, our perspective begins to change.

Healing can be done at various planes of existence. Every technique takes a unique approach in choosing the planes of existence for healing purposes. The ailment can begin on a subtle body and it can takes its own time to affect the physical body and be noticed at the physical level if timely and appropriate action is not taken to heal it at the root level.

While it is imperative that treatment and healing be done at the physical level, it is also necessary to try and get to the root cause of the ailment by working on subtle bodies of the individual. That brings the possibility to heal the ailment at the root level so that it does not propagate to physical level, beyond the level where it originated. Healing can also happen on multiple levels simultaneously.

The physical symptoms are an indication of something not going right at the subtle energy levels. Hence as soon as the symptoms start showing up, it is time to start working the physical level as well as the subtle levels to be able to deal with the ailment completely and effectively. It is recommended to consult one's physician before using alternative healing techniques. When we say "Time heals", it is understood to heal at all levels of existence, the physical, etheric, astral, mind and causal.

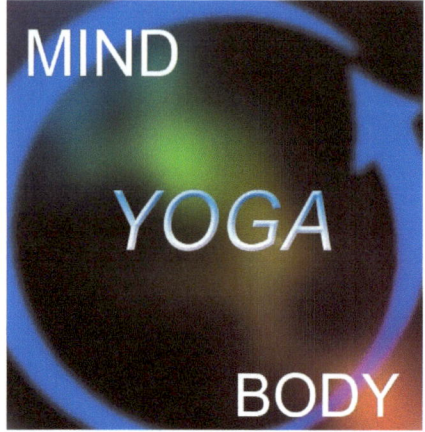

Yoga creates a circuit, a path for the inner energy to flow freely, and in the right manner so as to engender healing.

Yoga helps connect with the higher mind.

One of the goals of healing is the unification of conscious mind with the super consciousness, or the universal mind. Hence the name Yoga, or the union, as it interprets in Sanskrit language. Yoga can be practiced as a set of defined physical postures, for energy balancing, and it also refers to the techniques of meditation, Pranayama, sound healing, and several other healing techniques. It essentially refers to the method of unification of mind with the higher mind, and the method can be physical postures, or meditation, or energy work.

Chapter 3: Emotional Power

Emotions and feelings play a pivotal role in healing process and also in experiencing life as a whole. The feelings of joy, despair, elation, anger, jealousy, hatred etc. each of them carry a unique message for the individual who is experiencing them, and they are encoded for a certain purpose, in the individual's body and mind system.

The feelings of love, affection, and care provide solace, fulfillment and contentment to the mind and the soul. Emotional Intelligence is the key behind handling all one's feelings, and how they can be made to contribute towards the healing process. The world we sense with closed eyes is as real as the world we encounter with open eyes; however it exists in a different dimension.

There exists a lot of universe beyond the five senses that we often use while dealing with the world, and also with ourselves. Yoga and Meditation provide means and access to that inner dimension in our being, with comfort and ease, and help enhance the healing process.

Understanding both these worlds, the outer five-senses based world and the inner third-eye based world, interpreting them instinctively and intuiting leads to enhanced life awareness and handling of life events better. Based on the principles of energy healing, the places of worship have a collective healing energy around them, and they become like the energy base centers or healing centers and whoever comes in the vicinity of these centers, gets healed. Belief is a must to make these happen. Belief and Faith remove blocks in the pathways of mind body and soul healing.

The process of healing is multi-dimensional, and nature has provided us with great support and means to help us find one of the many of healing methods. Followed sincerely, one or more of these methods are sufficient for healing, while the energy healing process also takes into account, the Karma of the entities associated, and Unconditional love as energy is one of the greatest ways of healing the self as well as others.

The purer the love, the more power it has, as long as it is unconditional and given without any expectations in return. Blessings have immense healing power, preferably with no pre-conditions or expectations associated. Such expectations lead to Karma needing its own course of time and space to be cleared.

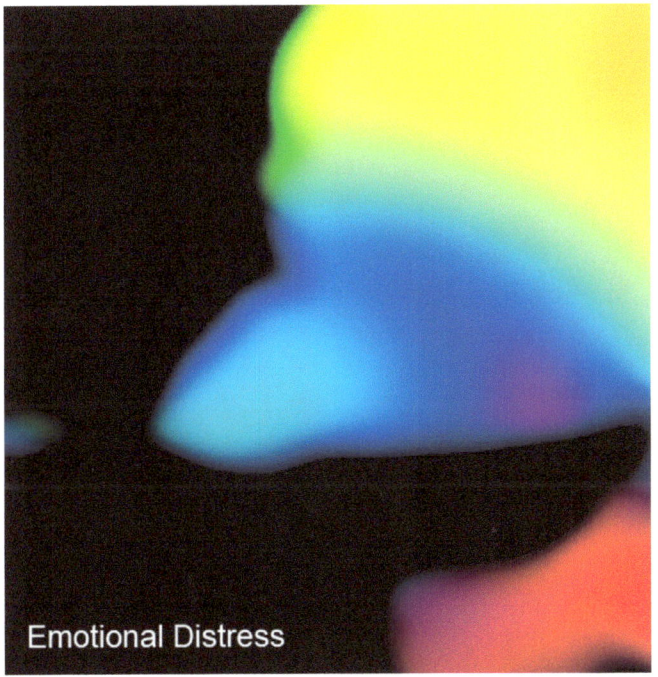

Emotional Distress

Emotional challenges can disturb the aura equilibrium

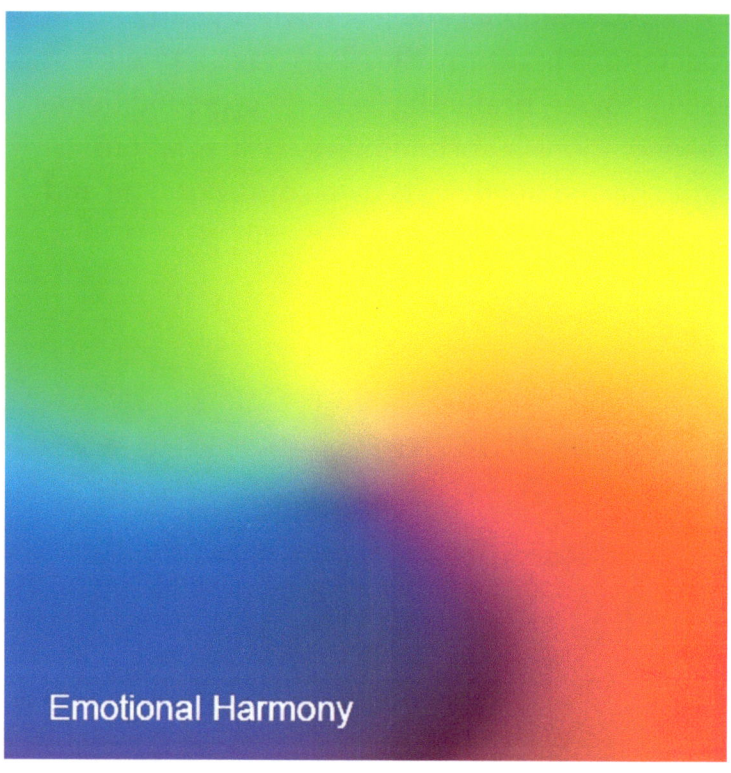

Emotional Harmony

The state of emotional harmony is determined by balanced colors in the individual's aura, and no blocks whatsoever in the emotional chakra, the solar plexus.

Chapter 4: Karma

Karma is generated every fraction of a second, if we were to measure it against time, but then it runs on many other dimensions and not just time. Time is just one of the factors. Spiritualists aim to become 'Karma Free' and work on not generating Karma, or rather Bad Karma, if you will. Buddha sat under a tree meditating for years and years, to attain Nirvana, moving towards Moksha, seeking freedom from life and death. Enlightenment, if interpreted as white light, appears to be a matrix of energies, emanating and moving towards light where light is the source and light, the destination. And we often end up saying, "Love and Light", as being part of healing session for self as well as others. In light, all identities disappear, all personalities disappear, and its soul and energy that remains.

Healing is an ongoing process, while it works on chronic energy patterns within the system; it also works on the day to day energy interactions, and hence works on past, present, and thus the future.

It is beyond time and space, and should preferably be done without any constraints in the mind to make it whole and complete.

Omnipresence, referring to the existence of an entity or soul, is a normal and natural phenomenon. It not only enables one's mind and soul presence at multiple places in longitude and latitude but also creates the opportunity of interacting with entities or people at multiple places. This happens for soul completion to continue to happen, gradually or sometimes rapidly moving towards its objective of achieving salvation or freedom or be free from bonds.

This also explains the process of astral projection, where mind leaves the body for an out-of-body experience to fulfill a task for higher good.

Every relationship is created by spiritual laws of attraction, and it lives until the interaction is whole and complete for highest good. The dynamics of the relationship work under the laws of Karma, and the goal is to fulfill the collective goal and set the souls free.

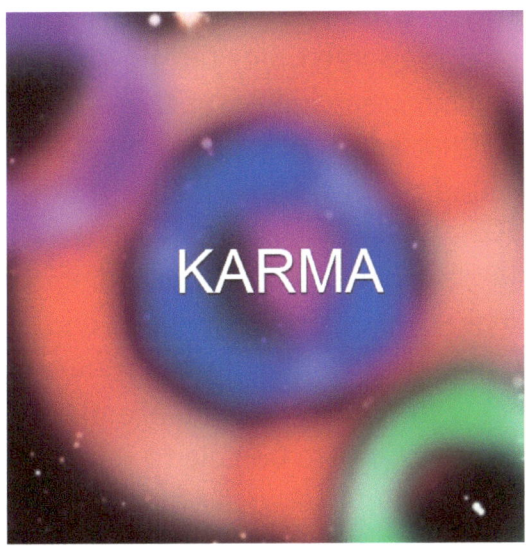

Karma is generated every moment across all dimensions

With Karma and its intricacies understood to some extent, the ways to heal are several and the doors to the destination are many. God continues to create several opportunities for the beings to connect with Him for higher guidance and direction enlightenment or soul awakening, He makes His presence felt from time to time, in so many ways, and we tend to address such situations as a 'co-incidence' or 'by chance happening', with nature at its creative best behind the scenes.

We are audience to a huge drama, a drama of reality so to say, where God makes us performs and project at the same time. Karmic transactions are created, chain reaction ensues, one thing leads to another, and another to another, and humans limited by their potential to memorize, can trace things back in a limited way, to a limited set of events, happening within limited time and space. And hence then arises the need and opportunity to surrender, listen to the inner self, and connect with the higher guidance, through the process of healing, to be able to see, hear, sense without the interference of the five senses. God then smiles a blessing.

Karma equations are complex, from what is known about him, even Gautama Buddha had tough time understanding Karma and spent several years understanding the process of Karma and dealing with it, before he could attain Nirvana. Karma can be understood as a cycle, a Karmic cycle so to say, and it is in relation to this, that we experience the fact that life goes full cycle. This full cycle is the Karmic cycle, and it is inescapable. The best to deal with it is to deal with it, and go through it, experience it with open heart, clear conscience, and honest mind.

Chapter 5: Time Dimension

Past, Present & Future exist all together, simultaneously in the spiritual world, the world that exists beyond science and the five senses. Time is essentially not linear, yet clocks and watches and now our computer clocks go on ticking so very regularly. Is life really that linear? Is it that regular? Then what significance does time have besides being a scheduling assistant? Linear measurement of time is vastly redundant. It is needed though. And it is needed at a very basic level. Beyond that basic level, time cannot help measure events and experiences that happen at various levels and planes of existence.

Time and pain are related in a nonlinear fashion. Pain determines destiny. The destiny that exists in the past, it exists in the present and in the future. Pain creates a path, a path to the destination, secretly coded in pain and its symptoms.

The path is treaded by initiating the process of healing the pain, or trying to get rid of the pain, where healing is a better choice over getting rid of it, since the second option is likely to sway the soul to experience another path of pain, possibly due to denial or non-acceptance of self-reality.

So if one follows the pain to its healing, learns from it, reads it, lives it to the extent possible, and it goes away, gets healed.

It is recommended to use healing methods, alternative or others to support the healing process, yet to heal it at the root level, natural ways of healing work better. Root cause of any pain or joy event can help trace one's individuality, soul nature and vibrations. But the process is tricky and it can succeed after years of practice on oneself.

Relating pain and joy to the time dimension, at any given time in one's life, the elements of past or present, that co-exist, would result from non-completion of the pain event or the joy event that happened in that past or in that present.
This becomes the start of the journey, the journey to learn from the pain or the joy event, and experience another bit of awareness.

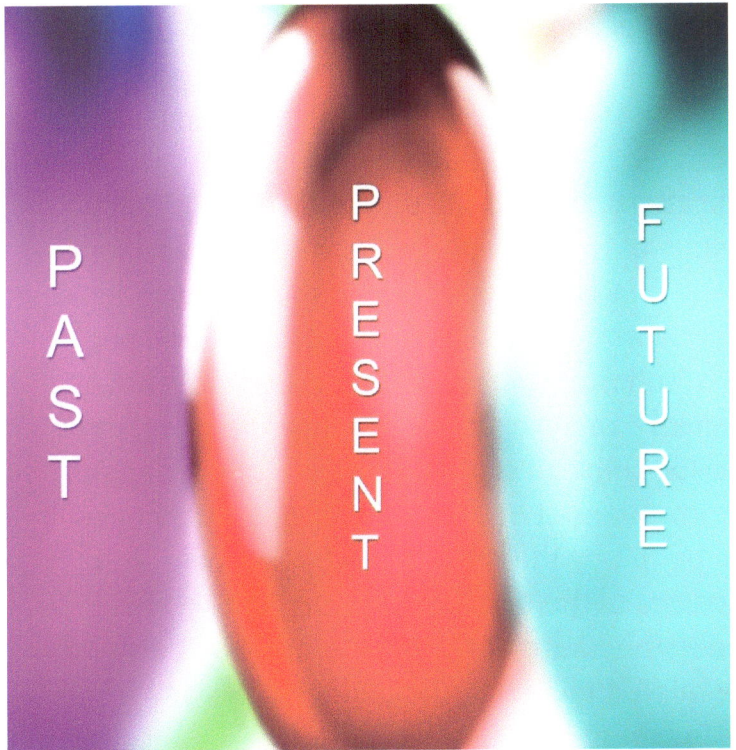

Isolating the past completely from present or future is tricky.

Even if these aspects are ignored during 'wide awake' time, they will linger on unless healed, and shall appear in form of entities in dreams, like shadows, or people, or thoughts

And this experience might even affect the physical self of the person, creating ailments. So it is essential that it is given priority to be healed and not taken lightly. Dreams provide signals, indications, path to the destination, forming the destiny of the individual. Silence has a story to tell, in fact an endless story, and one needs the right pair of ears to tune in, to connect and begin to listen to the sounds, noise or music. Translation of silence to a language one can understand does provide some clues, but there is a lot beyond it, and that cannot be represented in any language. It can be felt by the heart, even by the mind, and once again, the translated matter can be understood as a feeling for the heart and also for the mind, though mind is assumed to away from feeling matter and closer to logic.

The simultaneous existence of the being at several places in time and space has to understood and very delicately handled to handle life and healing. The limitations of the mind are unlimited, and life presents its complexities in infinite ways, whether it is to do with karmic associations, intricacies of events that happen, people playing numerous roles, and countless relationships one experiences on this planet.

An event at one place mysteriously affects another event at another location, leaving the subjects in a state of quandary and confusion. And hence the need to surrender to, 'Grace and Godliness' becomes unquestionably important. Trust on the instincts has to be complete in order to allow the healing to happen and allow the life to take its natural course.

Chapter 6: Yoga and Healing

Treat Yoga like an instrument, like a tool, a means to align your energy flow with the universal flow. Be it a Yoga position, a Yogic practice, a Mantra that is chanted, or a Meditation practice, these are all tools, methods, modalities, practices at physical, mental, emotional or spiritual level, that help one to move another step towards bliss and enlightenment. With continuous practice, dedication, and faith, any or all of these methods absolutely create positivity and abundance in life.

Choices can be made in life to bring about that desired change in life, but at the same time, the older patterns have to be healed, older relationships have to be healed whole and complete, so that the new set of choices can successfully bring about the desired change in life.

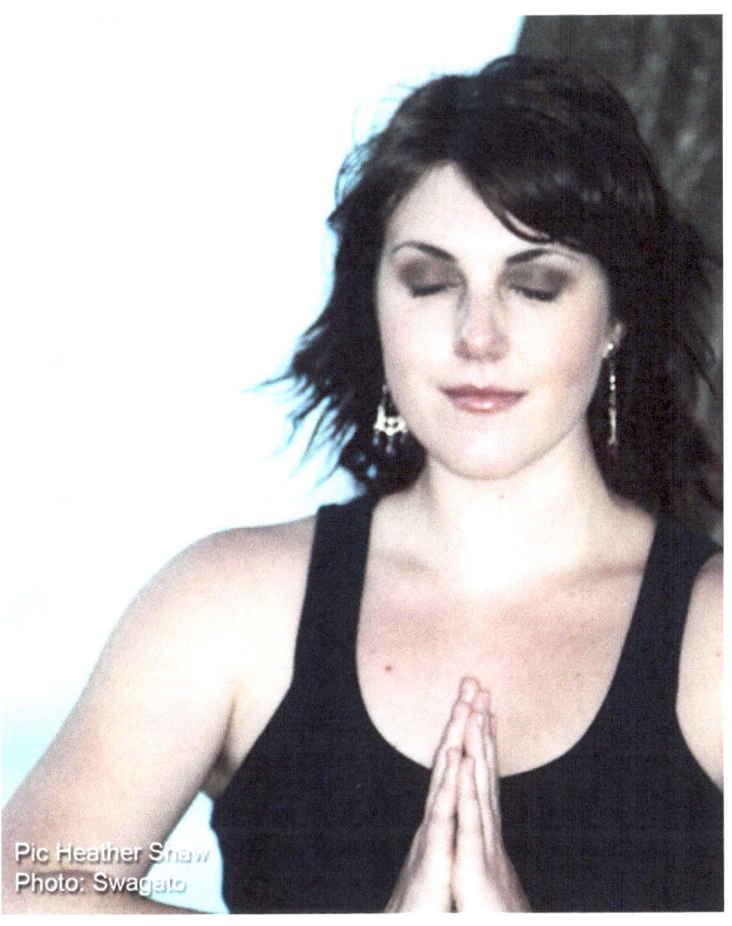

Pic Heather Shaw
Photo: Swagato

In rhythm with the super conscious mind

If not consciously, one always indulges in dealing with oneself subconsciously, and one's projection of others. These events and experiences also manifest as dreams sometimes in order for the healing process to be complete.

One interesting way to interpret one's own personality is to begin to understand what people mean to you, what their personalities look like to you, and how you begin you judge them based on your thoughts, beliefs and conditioning.
This is true for the good fact that you might discover them to be your own projections, the projections of your mind, or how you see them or how you want to see them. This is an interesting phenomenon and needs a lot of thought to be put into. There can be situations when without knowing the people and just merely looking at them or interpreting them from their appearance, cast, creed or sex, one can almost build their full character based one one's earlier experiences, beliefs and prior understanding of the society.

This often leads to wrong conclusions, misunderstanding, and invalid communication leading to more problems, and added complexities to one's life. Since in this experience, one is talking to or dealing with a projection of one's own self and not to the real being, in the other person. Even if there are moments of joy, and instant gratification and potential happiness in this experience, it is not likely to last long since there will be a time when the real personalities will clash, or rather interact, and masks will be removed, and projections will no longer be there. The key is deal with the world with open heart and open mind, and overcome the tendency to prejudge people just by their superficial persona. This process needs time, and with time, deeper bonds are created and relationships can be real and can last much longer. In cases where judgments have been made in the initial course of the relationship, there is still a possibility to come out of it, and make the relationship better. This can be accomplished by forgiveness, patience, and giving time and space to the person and to the relationship.

How about lost relationships and missed connections? Well, listen to your soul and listen to your heart, and see if you want to work on any of your lost relationships. If you do, heal them in your mind first, heal them in your heart first, and then see if there is an opportunity to get in touch with the people involved. If meant to be, rekindled love, and lost connections getting back in touch are not miracle situations. In today's world of social media networking, no one is really far away or lost if one really wants to make a connection, a good connection, an empowering connection!

Pain interpretation and experience varies from person to person, and pain, most of the time brings the messages from 'up there', acting as guides towards what actions need to be performed, as what 'medicines' have to be taken to get rid of that pain, or heal the pain, or heal the source of that pain. At times, it is not the pain that causes suffering, it's the meaning we associate with the pain experience translates pain as suffering or 'bad experience'.

Pain may occur for positive reasons, for betterment, for growth of the individual. Pain interpretation becomes difficult for the person who is in pain herself because as it happens is that during pain, the entire body attention is towards removing that pain. In those situations, taking outside support helps and the outside help has to be both trustworthy and reliable.

At times pain can be related to growth of the individual, physical, mental or both. In those situations, pain happens since the body or the mind is kind of adjusting to the new circumstances, coming out of previous comfort zone, or previous state, and is expanding in its ability to deal with these new circumstances. This is the time when blessings are needed, and God support is always there so that we are able to withstand the storm. As the body and the mind begin to adjust to the new state of existence, one feels more strength and power to be able to deal with life's tough experiences better. This needs one to stay surrendered to God, and get ego out of the way completely.

It may be easier than said, but it does help if one interprets all pain as opportunities and with gratitude and surrender, takes the actions that are righteous, true and in line with one's conscience. All this happens within the laws of Karma, and good karma is generated for righteous actions, where universal good is the intent, and no harm is meant for anyone.

Yoga works on the seven major Chakras found in the human body. These seven Chakras and their spinning, according to ancient spiritual sciences that have their roots in Indian ways of healing determine the state of the individual as being healthy or unhealthy. Food affects Chakras, Karma affects Chakras, and Thoughts affects Chakras. These Chakras are also found to be associated with each of our seven glands in the body. The root Chakra, at the base of the spine relates to our physical existence, and state of security.

The normal functioning of this chakra identified by color red, keeps us feel safe, secure about our physical state of existence, with our survival needs being met. The next Chakra, Hara Chakra, located below the navel relates to our sexual needs, and power of creativity. The normal functioning of this Chakra, identified by color orange, keeps us healthy in sexual realm, fully connected with our power of sexuality and creativity, free from doubts, guilt, and disempowering thoughts. The next Chakra, Solar Plexus Chakra is related to our emotions of joy, pain, despair, anger, jealousy, wants, passion, so on and so and so forth.

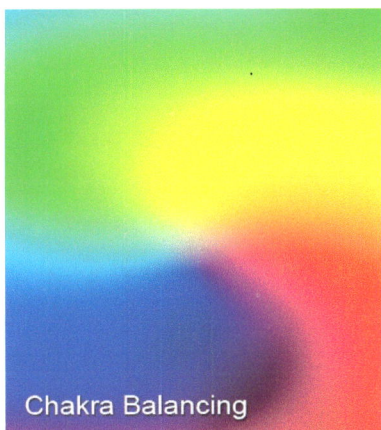

Chakra Balancing

Each Chakra is associated with a color, with a frequency, with a vibration

The emotions can empower or disempower people depending on how they respond to them, and what meanings they associate with them. If used well, emotional power can really contribute to making life a fulfilling journey.

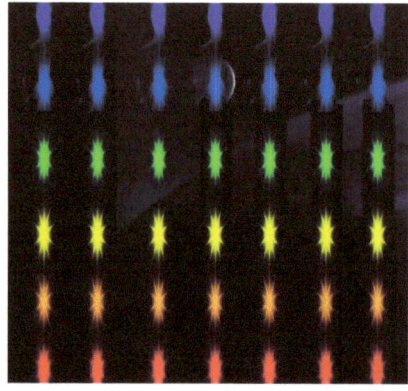

The seven colors associated with the Chakras

The normal functioning of this Chakra, associated with color yellow, helps one deal with emotions well, realizing the power of emotions, and making life experience fulfilling. The next Chakra, Heart Chakra is about unconditional love for oneself and others. The normal functioning of this Chakra, associated with color green transforms life into an extremely wonderful experience for the individual.

And since the Chakra is associated with selfless and unconditional love, there is never any despair or feeling of rejection since there are no expectations from the love that goes out to the world and the love that is experienced for oneself.

The next Chakra, Throat Chakra is about communication with oneself and others. The normal functioning of this Chakra, associated with color blue, enables one to communicate openly, truthfully, honestly and clearly with oneself and others. The next Chakra, Third Eye Chakra, is about clairvoyance, intuition, and sixth sense.

This Chakra, associated with color indigo helps connect one with the higher realms, higher guides, and energies to be able to see beyond time and space. The next Chakra, the last and major of the seven main Chakras, is called the Crown Chakra. This Chakra is divine Chakra and it connects the being to Godliness, and the super consciousness. The normal functioning of this Chakra, associated with color Violet, heals the connection of one's conscious mind, with the super conscious mind, the Godliness creating inner abundance for the individual!

The Chakras can be healed by Reiki, Pranayama Breath Yoga, by Color Healing, Crystals and several others ways of energy healing. Reiki is a powerful system of healing that utilizes specific techniques for restoring and balancing the natural life force energy within the body. It is a holistic, natural, hands-on energy healing system that touches individuals on all levels: body, mind, and spirit. The "Usui System" of Reiki Balances and strengthens the body's energy promoting its ability to heal itself. Besides the obvious use in serious illness, Reiki promotes the natural healing process in many other areas. Beyond the physical effects, Reiki also awakens the chakras, opening the individual to higher potentials. Various healing systems, including Reiki, which crossed many different cultures, emerged from this single root system.

As with many of the spiritual practices, and teachings of Tibet, these healing systems were a blend of both ancient oriental knowledge, as well as the teachings and wisdom of the yogic schools of ancient India.

Reiki is taught today, as it was in ancient times through a series of attunements, or transmissions, which can only be given to a student through a Reiki master.

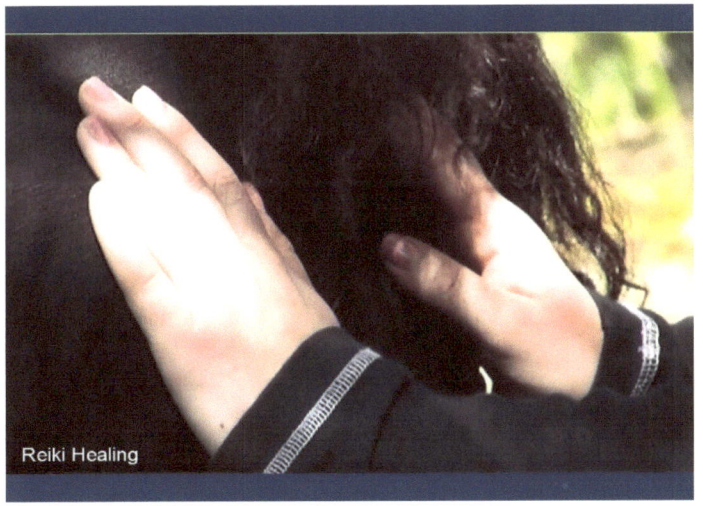

Reiki Healing

Reiki, as a pure form of divine life energy, flows through the entire being. Reiki Practitioners act as facilitators for this energy, which naturally flows to where it is most needed. For this reason, each individual's experiences of a Reiki Session happen at all levels of existence.

On the Physical Level, Reiki balances and replenishes the life energies of the physical body, aiding the process of healing. Reiki not only deals with the physical illness, however, but also the state of the soul.

On the Emotional Level, Reiki brings the higher self into connection with the personality, releasing emotional blockages, and bringing peace and harmony. Often deeply held emotional hurts, which color perceptions of reality are released during or after a Reiki Session, bringing the individual back to a more balanced emotional expression of self.

On the Spiritual Level, Reiki opens us up to the expression of our higher self, allowing us to discover all we can be, and the deeper meaning of life. As Reiki opens the various chakras, it also opens us to a deeper awareness of self, and often works as a catalyst for spiritual growth. Most people find that there is a marked improvement in there intuitive abilities after several sessions.

Those who undergo Reiki attunements also find that it works to awaken the various psychic abilities and spiritual virtues that are associated with the awakening of the various chakras.

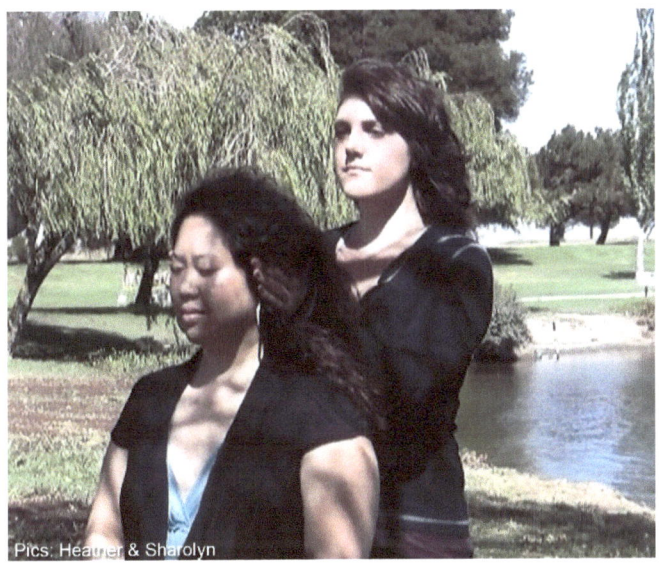

Pics: Heather & Sharolyn

Reiki healing session in progress

Another interesting aspect of Yoga is sound healing or sound therapy. Sound yoga is a technique in which sounds and vibrations are used to help restore, maintain, and improve one's state of mind and body. The Sanskrit word yoga is derived from the root yuj, meaning "to unite."

The music therapist uses the power of sounds to help clients improve their health, bringing a more positive state of mind, and enhancing their quality of life. The sounds create a multidimensional energy field, and help generate specific brain waves, resulting in shift in the state of consciousness of the person. The person then moves to a deep and relaxed state, the communication between mind, body, and spirit is enhanced, resulting in bliss. The healer, after diagnosis, chooses the appropriate sounds, to engender sound healing. Some healers use their voice, while others use Tibetan bowls, forks, flutes, chimes, didgeridoos, tanpura, and other instruments.

Every being vibrates within a range of frequencies, and when exposed to musical notes that match with the frequencies, it resonates with the note.

The healer has to bring the right frequencies, and vibrations in the vicinity of the person, to cause the state of resonance, thus engendering the move to a state of harmony.

Music can help overcome anxiety, enhance creativity and optimism. The human brain can be guided to come into resonance with the healthy vibrations. A stronger beat can stimulate the mind, with faster tempos helping to bring more focus, and a slower tempo creating a relatively tranquil state. Music can have a lasting influence on the state of mind, even after one has stopped listening to it. The Mozart Effect refers to the fact that some of Mozart's music has been found to cause more activity in certain areas of human brain.

With so many healing systems, and techniques available, at times it becomes a tough choice, which one to really choose and apply. Listen to your inner voice, connect with the inner mind, and see where it wants to take you. And then, have full faith in whatever choice you make, and the direction you choose. In a way, through your power of intuition, it is God who guides us all the time. Making multiple choices is an okay option to go for as long as one can manage them.

Eventually it is about removing the blocks within, in our mind, our body, our psyche and our consciousness. And as the blocks go away, giving way to clear energy flow, one begins to feel a shift in thinking, and an expansion of one's consciousness and aura presence. The consciousness is light, white light, encompassing and engulfing all colors of existence. "We are beings of light", is what is discovered in the process, and "We can be infinite" is what is understood in the whole experience.

An approach to enlightenment is to work on unifying the eternal polarities of existence, the male and the female, the Shiva and the Shakti. This unification is mental and spiritual rather than physical. This soul unification sparks off a light process, an experience of a lifetime. This energy can be used for creative purposes, and can guide one towards attaining the state of enlightenment. The process may be instantaneous, or may take several years and ages, depending upon how prepared the individuals are, to 'handle' the state of awakening and enlightenment.

Human mind and body have their limitations, and hence once triggered, the enlightenment process can take a lot of time till those limitations start diminishing and disappearing as one moves to a state of bliss, abundance and inner joy.

Chapter 7: Awakening

Awakening is a slow process; it cannot be sudden occurrence for a human being, it can bring a lot of energy onto the individual that can shake up one's system beyond control. And it relates to and is present in the past, the present and the future at the same time. There is a plane on which the past, the present, and the future connect to each other, and exist together, serving the individual. Meditation or any such 'delve into self' technique brings forth the past, the present, and the future at the same time to the meditator.

And there exists that choice for the meditator, to begin the healing process on oneself, by picking and selecting the events from that pool of life events, and begin the journey. Hypnotists do something similar, so do those who practice past life regression healing. Now that's another aspect – past life. For those who do not believe in the theory of reincarnation can conveniently categorize it under 'all the past' and then the applied concept is the same.

Dealing with the past, present and future at the same time. Another trick is to deal with joy or pain in the same way, and dealing with happiness or sadness in the same way. The understanding could begin by isolating oneself from the emotional states, and realizing the challenges that might exist in getting into the extreme states of joy or pain. But one has to know that if one indulges in joy in an extreme fashion, there may be a possibility that the next day, or the next phase, the state of pain, or 'non-joy' may become part of the experience and create a kind of emotional roller-coaster for the individual.

So if one is prepared to deal with the extreme situations, or experiences, it is fine to make them part of the life, but it would need a lot of energy, and balance for the individual to do so. Another approach is to take a mild stand with respect to the emotions, and keep oneself from the extremities. This is a safer approach, and helps one protect oneself from getting consumed by such extremities.

This can help the mind work better in stressful situations, where there probability of one getting consumed or overwhelmed is less and one can function better in society. A smart approach to managing the past, present and future events by an individual can help her succeed in living life the way she wants to, with a sense of completion experienced every day and every moment.

As one gets tempted to attain nirvana, awakening and enlightenment, there arises the need to leave the temptation away, and stay with the experience than to try to align with the outcome. Given the path is treaded sincerely and truthfully, awakening can never be far away, in fact the experience itself then becomes part of the awakening process, or the process of achieving enlightenment. And during the course itself, one can feel those glimpses of light, that are like an assurance from Godliness that yes, the path being treaded is right and taking one in the right direction towards the state of bliss.

Thank You

My biggest gratitude to God for giving me this opportunity to share my insight on the subjects of Karma, Yoga and Mind,, and my heartiest thanks to my family, friends, loved ones, and well-wishers for their continued support and motivation!

- Sandeep Khurana

info@skivamusic.com
http://facebook.com/sandeepkhuranaworldwide
http://youtube.com/sandeepkhuranas
http://twitter.com/sandeepkhurana

Relaxation and Meditation Music by Sandeep Khurana

Meditation and yoga are renowned for their positive impact both psychologically and physically, but it is best to truly relax to experience their full potential.

A calming backdrop of natural, soothing and calming songs and guides can create an environment perfectly tailored for the mind to shut out all thoughts of stress.

Their online store located at http://www.skivamusic.com features selected tracks composed by California based composer Sandeep Khurana till date.

His signature sounds are melodious, upbeat, rhythmic, uplifting, motivating, and energizing. Their new age music is based on the principles of Sound Yoga and Music Therapy, and the influence music can have on the minds of listeners.

Music shoppers can download the latest in Guided Meditations, Reiki Music, Chants, Easy Listening, World Fusion and Workout music from SK Infinity.

These sounds and vibrations tend to create an invisible multidimensional energy field and healing environment, helping create specific brain waves, resulting in complete shift in the state of consciousness of the person. The person then moves to a deeper and relaxed state, the communication between mind, body, and spirit is enhanced, resulting in bliss.

Sandeep Khurana has been creating compositions for relaxation since 2007 with over 100 albums now on iTunes for both meditation and fitness music. His style of New Age, with Fusion and a pinch of Healing Music, have taken him to the being ranked in the top 100 New Age artists in iTunes, as well as his music featuring on Spotify and Rhapsody.

Sandeep Khurana's music, also available for streaming on popular radio channels like Pandora radio and Sky.fm, has received tremendous response from listeners worldwide, with the subscriber base crossing a million in over 50 countries, and more than 60 of its tracks figuring in iTunes Top 100 New Age Music Charts worldwide.

The SK Infinity Music online store at http://skivamusic.com offers a great collection of Sound Yoga and Music Therapy tracks for downloads.

The store features secure shopping with payments accepted through PayPal, Google Checkout and major credit cards.
For details, please visit http://music-mantra.com and http://skivamusic.com

Mantras for Empowerment

Lord Ganesha

Om Gama Ganapataye Namaha

Lord Shiva

Om Namaha Shivaya

Gayatri Mantra

Om Bhurbhuvasvaha Tatsaviturvarenyam
Bhargodevasyadhimahi Dhiyoyonaprachodayaat

Lord Brahma (Guru Mantra)

Gurubrahma Guruvishnu Gurudevo Maheswarah
Guru Saakshaat Param Brahma Tasmai Shri
Guravey Namaha

Lord Shani

Om Shri Shanaishcharaaya Namaha

Lord of the Universe

Om Namo Bhagavate Vasudevaya

Lord Krishna and Lord Rama

Hare Krishna Hare Krishna Hare krishna Hare Hare
Hare Rama Hare Rama Rama Rama Hare Hare

"AUM"